LIFE WITH RHEUMATOID ARTHRITIS

ROSS LENNOX

INTRODUCTION FROM THE AUTHOR

In 2014 I was finally diagnosed with the debilitating condition of rheumatoid arthritis. The diagnosis took a long time coming, as did any form of medication to counter the condition, and as a result I spent eight months of my life near enough on the sofa at home. I could not walk without crying, my knees and ankles were so badly swollen I could barely get my jeans on and I had no chance of getting any shoes on and I was forced to wear slippers. It is an all too familiar situation for those people unfortunate to suffer from the disease.

During this eight month period when I was existing on concoctions of steroids and pain killers I read every single article I could find on rheumatoid arthritis.

Although the final diagnosis took a long time in coming every medical practitioner I saw and every nurse was fairly sure that I did indeed had RA.

During this time it became painfully obvious to me, apologies for the pun, that I was suffering from a western condition brought about by my diet. If you had asked me about my diet before I was diagnosed with RA I would have told you I had a pretty healthy diet. Plenty of fish, loved my smoothies and juices - but I also loved cakes, take away and eating out. So although I did have plenty of healthy food I was also having plenty of unhealthy food, or at least enough to tip the scales in favour or RA.

The more I read the more I had to question what on earth was going on. It seems that the first recorded case of RA in

Africa was in the 1960's even though the disease had been around in Europe and recognised since the late 1800's. And that was another thing - it's a new disease, where did it come from? What was causing it? It is also virtually unknown it appears in countries like South America and Asia, and this made me start to wonder what made me so different from the people in those countries. The answer was of course very simple, diet.

Post my diagnosis I was on a fairly awful set of drugs. Methotrexate was one of these. The drug is I believe is one that they use in chemo-therapy. I would take this, along with a few other drugs on Monday, and I cannot begin to describe how tired it made me feel. I was dogged with a lethargy I just could not shake until about Thursday/Friday when finally I felt a little more alive and motivated, and then all too soon again it was Monday and I would be back at the bottom again. Along with the tiredness were other unpleasant side effects like constant head aches and mouth ulcers. The steroids I had been taken had the unwanted side effect of making me have an over active appetitive, that coupled with the inactivity of sitting on the sofa soon saw the pounds pile on.

This book will also help you understand how the immune system and its inflammatory mechanism work. The immune system is a vital part of the body that helps to protect us from injury and disease, but sometimes it goes haywire and creates problems instead, such as in the case of rheumatoid arthritis. Fortunately, there are many remedies available, and an anti-inflammatory diet is one of them. Read on to find out how you can adopt an anti-inflammatory diet. Know what foods to avoid because they cause inflammation, and what foods to eat more of to reduce the symptoms of inflammation. An understanding of what Rheumatoid Arthritis actually is becomes a necessary part of your new life. I found that information and the few leaflets I was provided with were woefully inadequate and I was left with many questions.

I wish you all the best of luck and hope that this book will provide you with some answers to help you along with you new life journey.

Ross Lennox

<u>Arthritis</u>

Arthritis is a common disorder but is not clearly understood. It's actually not a single disease, this term is commonly used to represent joint pain or joint related diseases. A joint is the site where two bones meet. For example, hip joint, where the femoral head (thighbone) meets the acetabulum (pelvis); knee joint, where tibia and fibula two bones meet, the bones of lower leg. In medical sciences, there are above hundred types of such conditions. Cartilage covers the end of the bones and cushions them and allows joints to move easily by lubricating them, reducing friction. Joints are covered by fibrous envelope (synovium), a fluid that helps in friction reduction as well. Ligaments and tendons help the joints of muscles with bones to stabilize. Tendons give them power and allow the bones to move. Arthritis affects people of all ages, races and sexes, and it's a prominent cause of disability all over the world. It is very common among females and older people.

Common symptoms of arthritis include stiffness, swelling, decreased range of movement and pain. These symptoms may appear and disappear, can be sever, moderate or mild. Some symptoms remain the same for the long term and some may progress and worsen over the passage of time. Lupus arthritis or rheumatoid arthritis is caused as a consequences of a systemic disease in whole body. Inflammation is the body's normal reaction as in rheumatoid arthritis, but the consequences can be severe enough to cause permanent disability.

Rheumatoid Arthritis

Rheumatoid arthritis is a common autoimmune disorder in which a person's own immune system – the defensive mechanism of the body that normally attacks foreign substances e.g. viruses and bacteria, mistakenly starts to attack the joints, causing severe joint inflammation. This causes the tissue lining present inside of joints (synovium) to thicken, resulting pain and swelling of the joints. Synovium produces fluid to lubricate the joints for smoother working, reducing friction. If the condition remains untreated for a long time, it can damage cartilage, the soft tissue layer that protects the ends of bones and joints. During the passage of time, the individual can suffer from cartilage loss and the spacing between bones becomes reduced and joints become painful, unstable, loose and lose their mobility.

Because of irreversible joint damage, healthcare specialists recommend early diagnosis and rapid treatment to overcome rheumatoid arthritis. Rheumatoid arthritis mainly affects the bones and joints of wrist, ankles, feet, elbows, knees and hands. It is a systemic disorder which means if the one hand or knee is affected, commonly the other one is also affected. Rheumatoid arthritis also affects other body systems as well, e.g. respiratory, skin, eyes or cardiovascular system. It is called systemic disease, meaning it is related to whole body.

Some environmental and genetic factors affect the possibility of being diagnosed with rheumatoid arthritis. According to a recent survey, a family history i.e. parents or grandparents suffering from rheumatoid arthritis, increase the chances of this disorder by about three to five times. Genomic studies have found that about 100 genes are associated with the risk of rheumatoid arthritis; other mutations and innate immunity (general defensive mechanism, present from birth) also influence the occurrence of rheumatoid arthritis. Some environmental risk factors e.g. smoking, silica exposure and excess alcohol consumption also increase the chances of rheumatoid arthritis but according to another study low alcohol consumption may have positive influence as it may provide protective. There is another disorder known as periodontal disease; involving the infection in ligaments or tissues present in bones.

<u>Being diagnosed with rheumatoid arthritis</u>

This disorder is basically different for everyone. You may have different signs/ symptoms from other rheumatoid arthritis patients, and it may not follow an identifiable pattern. Symptoms may appear early, only overnight; or they may appear gradually including months or years so that it's difficult to pinpoint when they began. It is also difficult for a healthcare specialist to establish what sort of joint disorder you are dealing with, prior to confirmation that it is rheumatoid arthritis. It is hard to diagnose because a few symptoms of this disease can appear in other diseases, for example painful and swollen joints may be due to some bacterial or viral infections.

To make a diagnosis, healthcare specialists consider a combination of things e.g. your history: the various symptoms you've ever suffered with. These may comprise joint pain, the feeling of being tired even after a little work, joint stiffness, especially in the morning and other flu-like symptoms. Any family history of this disease or other similar conditions. There will be examinations of affected joints, and a rheumatologist will generally make blood tests. There is no particular blood test that can tell us exactly about arthritis, but commonly rheumatoid arthritis patients have symptoms of inflammation in their body fluids like blood: the presence of particular antibodies (designated as "anti-CCP" and "rheumatoid factor"). Medical imaging of your joints to visualize the symptoms of damage or inflammation. Imaging may be magnetic resonance imaging (MRI), x-rays or ultrasound scans.

After diagnosis of rheumatoid arthritis, you should discuss the options with your healthcare specialist and start the advised treatment as it will be the start of you having some control on your rheumatoid arthritis.

Feelings after diagnosis with rheumatoid arthritis

Being diagnosed with rheumatoid arthritis is frequently tough to come to terms with. This news maybe a shock or a relief, many people find it a helpful to know what's wrong and what can they do to treat this disease. Whatever your feelings are, you don't need to deal with this on your own. One of the most critical things is to have a person to talk to about your situation. Friends and family members can help to support you. Healthcare professionals are there to give valuable advice to prevent and reduce your symptoms.

Conversations with other patients experiencing rheumatoid arthritis can also be helpful as they can often understand your situation. You may feel irritated because this has happened to you, or may you want to ignore it. It is absolutely normal to have these sort of strong feelings. It is also entirely normal to get annoyed if you can't do whatever you want to, also it is difficult to accept help from others if you never had it before. Some people understandably start worrying about their future and feel they should start to manage better.

You may find your eyes become blurry and light sensitivity. Long term inflammation cause also scaring in your lungs and heart tissues, causing chronic dry coughs and a shortness of breath. During some severe cases, people may develop nodules in lungs or abnormal lung tissues because of high inflammation that can be only be seen by x-rays. These nodules are commonly benign and range in various size from small pea like lumps to ones as large as a walnut. In majority of cases they don't cause pain.

According to a recent survey more than 80% of rheumatoid arthritis patients say they always feel tired and fatigued. This number increases when we talk about a combination of disorders e.g. headache, depression and obesity. You may feel unwell or tired even after a long rest even early in the morning not long after getting up. The difficulty in getting out of bed or walking in the morning due to pain and stiffness in your ankles, feet or knees can tire you out. This stiffness generally is severely bad during morning and may last about 45 minutes to an hour.

When you feel better, people with rheumatoid arthritis are encouraged to do some healthy aerobic exercise e.g. walking or light workouts to improve your muscular strength. This will lower the pressure on your joints and improve your overall health. An occupational or physical therapist can prove helpful to find the activities that are best suited to your body condition. Thanks to highly improved current modes of treatments, all the negative feelings start decreasing when you have your strength and energy back and have relief from the stiffness and pain in your joints. You should also talk about these feelings with your healthcare specialist and other people who are victim of this disorder.

How does rheumatoid arthritis affect you?

When people talk about arthritis or rheumatoid arthritis, they generally consider it as an older person's disease related to joint damage. They are probably thinking about osteoarthritis or correlating these two types of arthritis. Rheumatoid arthritis is a totally different term. It is an auto-immune disorder as previously described in which your body's own defensive mechanism starts to act against your body and begins to damage the protective layer present around the bones end and joints. Our immune system is a complicated protective mechanism comprising antibodies and other cells to protect us from infectious diseases. Normally, it attacks things having harmful effect on our body. Inflammation is basically a healthy response of the body to protect itself from incoming infection. During a rheumatoid arthritis flare the body's own tissues and cells are attacked by the immune system, especially the lining of joints, resulting in painful, inflamed and swollen joints.

If you are a smoker, you should quit that worthless idea after being diagnosed with rheumatoid arthritis because smoking can decrease the effectiveness of your medications and slows the body's mechanisms to deal with some drugs. Also, this disease has worse outcomes in smokers as compared with non-smoking persons. In the modern era, the treatment has improved and its possible for you to lead an active life with this condition, the major thing is to take your prescribed medications in time and make some necessary daily life work changes.

You must keep in mind that it is a prolonged condition and not related to old age and people can develop rheumatoid arthritis at any stage of life even from childhood. For the majority of people, symptoms usually begin to appear between age 40 to 60 years. Moreover, there is no defined pattern of symptoms of this disease as everybody suffers in different ways. On top of stiffness, joint pain and swelling, some people may feel intensely tired, face difficulty in sleeping also feel like they have severe flu. It doesn't affect joints only but also influences other parts of the body like the lungs and eyes. If left untreated rheumatoid arthritis can cause sever joint damage if inflammation remains uncontrolled for a long time. It's a progressive disorder but its development varies from individual to individual. Early diagnosis and accurate treatment of this disease can control the future complications and allow people to spend whole of their lives normally with their symptoms under control.

<u>Symptoms of rheumatoid arthritis</u>

The major symptoms are joint swelling, stiffness, redness and warmth. On top of these main symptoms, others include poor appetite, high fever or temperature, dry eyes, lack of energy or tiredness, sweating, and chest pain. This disorder can damage any joint of the body, though, it is frequently noticed among the smaller joints in the feet and hands first. This is systemic as both sides of the body generally suffer in same way at the same time, but it is not an essential rule. Some people during this disease grow fleshy lumps commonly designated as rheumatoid nodules, around affected joints under the skin. In some cases, they can cause severe pain but are not commonly painful.

Extreme fatigue may be a sign of presence of anemia or thalassemia, lack of healthy red blood cells. Your healthcare specialist should examine you properly using blood tests as a part of their essential diagnosis methods.

Depression is also another prevalent symptom sufferers also have to deal with. This chronic disorder is difficult to live with. Rheumatoid arthritis can affect the lining of lungs. This is known as pleurisy and it can lead to shortness of breath. This can be treated by some pharmacotherapies suggested by your doctors. Like the lungs, damage can occur to the lining of heart muscles basically known as pericarditis or myocarditis. Its symptoms may also not appear, but it may lead you to suffer chest pain and shortness of breath and discomfort. This can also increase other cardiac complications such as heart failure, stroke and arterial fibrillation.

Rheumatoid arthritis may cause your eye-sight to weaken or cataracts to form leading to clouding of the lens. Scleritis is another eye related disorder also known as the redness of the white portion of the eye, this may also be due to inflammation. The damage to tear glands can also take place in severe cases leading to the improper tear film formation on the eyes, commonly known as dry eye syndrome. During rheumatoid arthritis a person may get a syndrome known as Sjogren's syndrome causing dryness in your mouth, eyes and inside of your nose. Kidneys and liver are rarely affected but the medications including nonsteroidal anti-inflammatory drugs (NSAIDs) are harmful for both organs. For example, methotrexate can cause liver damage, while cyclosporine is a cause towards kidney failure. Moreover, these drugs slow down your immune system and make you susceptible to major bacterial and viral infections.

Symptoms can be severe enough to cause paralysis or sudden death when the nervous system is attacked. This can be the consequence of joints damage during rheumatoid arthritis, medications used for the treatment and/or the disease process itself. Another may be the inflammation of blood vessels, these can look like spots on the skin.

Limping from decreased lower back functions can lead towards many diseases of nerves, bones and muscles of the lower extremities. It frequently occurs when arthritis affects the feet, knees, ankles and hips. Fever is also noticed among rheumatoid arthritis patients. Typically, it is a mild condition, rapidly corrected when the inflammation is controlled in the body. Because patients have to take medications to decrease the immune attack to the joints, it is significant as when they develop fever, the inflammation is a possible cause. A rapid treatment is required to control this inflammation.

Causes of rheumatoid arthritis

Healthcare specialists know a great deal about the consequences of rheumatoid arthritis and also about the treatment of this disease, but they also have not enough knowledge yet about what causes this disease in first place. Clinical studies so far indicate several combined factors may cause rheumatoid arthritis. Genetics play a great role in its pathogenesis, though is not essential that a child will definitely have rheumatoid arthritis if his or her parents are suffering from rheumatoid arthritis. Few genes make a person more susceptible to the progression of rheumatoid arthritis, though it is not an inevitable fact. When someone possess these genes in their genome, what sort of elements are required to trigger the arthritis process? It is not clear yet what these "triggers" actually are, but biomedical scientist suggests that stress, cigarette smoking, poor diet, injury or some sort of viral infection may play a part.

During the previous decade, new fields of research have opened up. Several mode of biological treatments are available including therapies targeting various aspects of bodies immune system causing tissue inflammation. There are a whole host of drugs available to help combat the disease, such as sulfasalazine, methotrexate leflunomide and hydroxychloroquine. Several clinical studies are being conducted to investigate the effects on the immune system and in the future these may provide different methods of treatment or even a cure.

Obesity or being overweight is a significant cause of rheumatoid arthritis in the young population. If you are overweight, your chances of developing rheumatoid arthritis increase 3-4 fold as compared with people with a normal body mass index (BMI). BMI is the measurement of weight compared with height and weight. For an adult person, a normal BMI could be in the range of 18.5 – 24.9. A few clinical studies also present great deal of evidence that consumption of too much red meat and the little or no intake of vitamin C in your diet also increase the risk of rheumatoid arthritis. Hormones may have a great influence on the pathophysiology of rheumatoid arthritis as well as it is more common in females as compared with males, this may be the influence of estrogen, this link has not been proven by any scientific studies, but it surely occurs more in males. Muscle trauma is also an independent cause of rheumatoid arthritis.

Mental and physical stress is also one of these. The mechanism is not clearly defined, but a common belief is that excessive and sudden release of stress hormones e.g. adrenaline and cortisol may influence the autoimmune response. The response of the body to physical stress reflects the response of this phenomena to emotional stress. While scientific studies are being conducted to evaluate the exact relationship of rheumatoid arthritis and mental stress, people facing this disorder often experience flare-ups, led by excessive depression, anxiety and fatigue.

Other triggers may be the flu and cold, which are also involved in immune system activation. Flare-ups can also be a symptom after consumption of a particular food triggering an allergic response. Some recent psychological studies are also available that suggest difficulties at work and breakup in a relationship, divorce and increase in financial obligations also have a negative impact on health and can serve as a potential trigger for rheumatoid arthritis.

Recent clinical studies also suggest there is a link between periodontal gum disease and rheumatoid arthritis. So, a regular dental checkup is also necessary. Just keep in mind that early treatment can cause your symptoms to be less severe and prevent your bones and joints from getting damaged. Ideally, you should start to treat disease within first 3 to 6 months.

About your care while living with rheumatoid arthritis

What sort of services are being provided varies, depending on your local healthcare. Whatever the services available, various healthcare professionals with particular knowledge related to rheumatoid arthritis will be involved in your care. You may visit to few of them regularly for proper treatment and be referred to others when required.

Wear such clothes that remain comfortable and easy to wear and remove from the body. Always go to your doctor with your previous history including complementary medicines and supplements, so that your rheumatology team can understand your situation exactly. Clearly describe your situation, tell them how you've been, even if you are currently not experiencing the symptoms. The clearer the team are about your condition the better understanding they will have about you; the better suggestions will be given as to your care plan.

Keep a diary to write daily levels of fatigue and pain as it could be helpful for your healthcare team. Clear everything with your doctor, ask any questions you want to even if you consider some to be silly, they won't consider them as such, and the more answers you have the better.

Balanced work and rest

During severe joint pain or swelling, you may be advised to take complete bed rest as your body won't allow you to do work. Try not to bed rest for more than one or may be two days. Spending extra time, laying on the sofa or bed may increase your body stiffness and start join pain. Once you feel little bit relief, get up and walk, stretch you body and continue your routine activities. You don't need to cut yourself off from other, you need to strike a balance between work and exercise, and recognize that on some days you may be able to do either. Tell your friends and family about your condition and let them understand that you need their help and support. Manage expectations for yourself. Rather than working to make a meal for friends, just invite them to your home and order pizza. Getting together for refreshment and conversation not just for food.

Eat well

During severe pain in rheumatoid arthritis you may loose your appetite and you may not have enough energy to prepare a meal by yourself. But a healthy balanced diet is crucial, you need a diet full of nutrition. This is especially so when your condition is poor as nutrition will work as a fuel for your body to produce heat. Moreover, eating a plenty of fresh vegetables and fruits, cold water fish (salmon), whole grains and lean meats which are all rich in omega-3 fatty acids, have a positive role in the fight against inflammatory cells. Also, it may be helpful for you to have small amount of food after short periods of time rather than eating a big meal. Avoid tobacco, alcohol, sweets and processed foods.

A little bit of chocolate can help you to manage your healthy diet plans during rheumatoid arthritis. There are certainly times when desserts or any sort of comfort food are just the things to boost your spirits.

<u>Try cold and heat</u>

Cold is better for acute pain relief and swelling. Use ice bags or the bags of frozen vegetables and cover them in a towel. Place 15 minutes on the area where the swelling is and then remove for 15 minutes and repeat the process. Heat can relieve stiffness and aches by elevating blood flow in muscles and relaxing them. You can try warm baths, heat pads or hot compresses.

<u>**Relieve stress**</u>

Anxiety and stress can make your condition even worse. Guided imagery, hypnosis, muscle relaxation, deep berating exercise, tai chi, yoga or visualization can help relief pain. You can also relive anxiety or stress by talking with family or with a friend, writing in a journal, taking part in a support group or engaging in a peaceful hobby i.e. gardening. An acupuncture or a massage can help relieve the stress and pain. Use your strong muscles for working where possible e.g. pick up your grocery bag on forearm rather than holding it with your fingers

<u>Use pain reliving medications</u>

Medicines like ibuprofen, acetaminophen, or naproxen sodium can be helpful for pain relief caused by rheumatoid arthritis. But make sure you consult your health care specialist before taking these medications. Your prescription for rheumatoid arthritis may differ and these may provide harmful to you, or stop other medication from working, so it is always best to check.

When you should call the doctor

If you feel severe pain caused by cold or due to overexertion, it is probably okay, and there is no need to worry overly. Practice self care tips and wait for a couple of days to see if there is an improvement. You should call the healthcare specialist in cases where you don't improve in a few days. If your condition is worsened because you forgot to have your medications properly, just pick the phone and talk to your doctor because both of you need a new plan for getting you back on track.

Medications/ drugs available for rheumatoid arthritis

Several drugs are available on the market for the betterment of this disorder, you can have these medications but remember one thing, consult your doctor for a proper understanding of your body's situation and other biochemical processes so that you do not harm your body. A few of these drugs are discussed below:

Steroidal drugs

Prednisone is a corticosteroid drug, that reduces the joints inflammation and pain and provides relief from joint damage.

Side effects may include diabetes, rapid weight gain and thinning of the bones. Healthcare specialists often suggest corticosteroid for the treatment of acute rheumatoid arthritis.

Disease modifying antirheumatic drugs

Commonly known as DMARDs, the drugs that can reduce the progression rate of this autoimmune disorder and save tissues and joints from prolonged damage. The main DMARDs are methotrexate (e.g. Rasuvo, Otresxup, Trexall), hydroxychloroquine (e.g. Plaquenil),leflunomide (e.g. Arava) and sulfasalazine (Azulfidine). Side effects may include lung infection, severe liver damage or bone marrow suppression.

Biological agents

This is an emerging group of DMARDs also known as bio response modifiers, including adalimumab (Humira),certolizumab (Cimzia), golimumab (Simponi),rituximab (Rituxan),tofacitinib (Xeljanz), abatacept (Orencia),anakinra (Kineret),etanercept (Enbrel),infliximab (Remicade) and tocilizumab (Actemra). These drugs have become increasingly effective when used in combination with other nonbiological DMARDs like methotrexate. These medications can target part of the immune system and trigger inflammation causing tissue and joint damage.

Alternative bio based medicines

Plant oils

The seeds of black currant, borage and evening primrose have omega-3 type fatty acids that are helpful in treating joint stiffness and pain in rheumatoid arthritis. The side effects may include diarrhea, nausea and gas. Some plant oils interfere with drugs and also can cause liver damage, so consult with your doctor first.

Fish oil

Some research studies have found the effectiveness of fish oil against rheumatoid arthritic inflammation, pain and stiffness.

Side effects may be fishy taste and bleaching. Fish oils also can interfere medications, so first consult with your doctor and follow their advice.

Orthopedic Surgery

If the drugs fail to treat and prevent joint damage, you and your rheumatology team may find the last possible option to be surgery to repair damaged joints. Orthopedic surgery can help you to regain your ability to move and use joints in a proper way. It can correct deformations and reduce pain. Surgery does come with a risk of pain, infection and bleeding. Other risk factors you should discuss with your healthcare specialists. Surgery for treatment of rheumatoid arthritis may involve following procedures:

Tendon repair

Inflammation by rheumatoid arthritis may loosen and rupture your tendons and damage the joints. Your surgeon may repair your tendons.

Synovectomy

Surgery involving the removal of damaged lining of the joints (synovium) can be performed on hips, elbows, fingers, knees and wrists.

Overall joint replacement surgery

Surgeon may eliminate the injured part of your joints and add a plastic, prosthesis made, or metal joint instead.

Joint fusion surgery

Surgical fusion of joints to realign or stabilize a joint for relief from joint pain may be a good option when joint replacement is not an option.

Conclusion

Rheumatoid arthritis affects about 0.5 to 1.0 % of the total adult population in developed countries. This percentage is increasing rapidly by on average, 100,000 per year with a highly growing rate. The rheumatoid arthritis development rate is 3 to 5 times higher in women as compared to men.

Rheumatoid arthritis currently has no cure and also people suffering from this disease don't present constant symptoms rather they present symptoms of severe flare-ups followed by symptom free periods designated as remission periods. The progress of arthritis can vary from person to person and time to time even in same individual and its symptoms can vary from mild to severe. Early treatment is essential to have a better quality of life. There is much you can do to live a happy life even with this debilitating disease.